Butterfly Kisses and Wishes on Wings

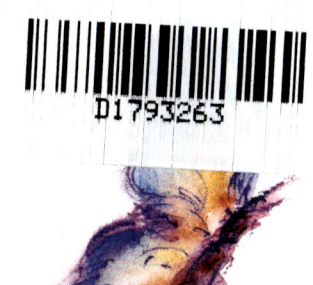

When someone you love has cancer
... a hopeful, helpful book for kids

Written by Ellen McVicker
Illustrated by Nanci Hersh

Butterfly Kisses and Wishes on Wings is a gem. This is a very important book with a very powerful message. A beautiful work of art that educates children about medical and psychological issues relating to cancer, it is also a gift for the loved one with cancer. As the public television personality Doc Neil the Banana Peel, I have had the opportunity to perform for kids and adults with cancer to help them relax and enjoy life. For a patient with cancer, there is no better gift than the comforting words and hugs from a kid who understands … it brightens the day. ***Butterfly Kisses and Wishes on Wings*** provides a pathway to this gift.

Neil Shulman, MD, author of *What's in a Doctor's Bag?*
Associate professor, Emory University School of Medicine
Author and associate producer, "Doc Hollywood" starring Michael J. Fox
President, Patch Adams' Gesundheit! Institute

A portion of the proceeds to benefit cancer research and education.

All rights reserved.

Text copyright © 2006 by Ellen McVicker
Illustrations copyright © 2006 by Nanci Hersh

No part of this book may be reproduced or used in any form or by any electronic or mechanical means, including information storage and retrieval systems, without permission in writing from the author, except in the case of brief quotations embodied in critical articles and reviews.

ISBN 978-0-578-15993-5

Book design and production by Fran Waldmann, fswaldmann@gmail.com
Production services provided by Manahawkin Printing, Athens, GA (706) 395-4874
Printed in Canada
1st Printing September 2006
2nd Printing January 2007
3rd Printing January 2009
4th Printing July 2010
5th Printing July 2012
6th Printing - First Paperback Edition March 2015
7th Printing May 2018
8th Printing February 2021

www.butterflykissesbook.com

Dedication

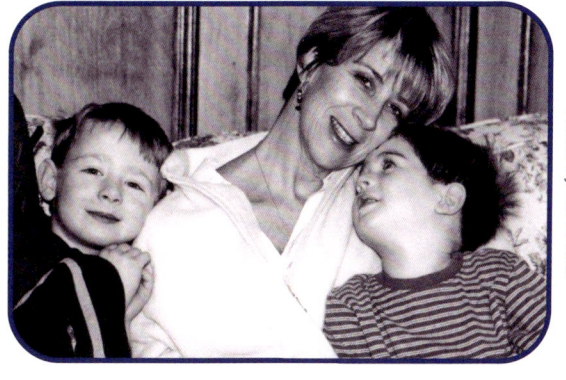

Photo by Terri Blair

This book is lovingly dedicated to my cousin Nanci Hersh's sons, Griffin and Nate who, when ages 5 and 3, put on ***their*** butterfly wings so they too could travel with their mom through her cancer journey.

And in loving memory of two remarkable visionaries...

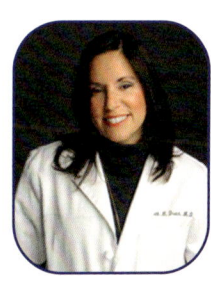

Dr. Beth Deutch
Founder of **HerSpace**, a Breast Imaging and Biopsy Center serving Monmouth and Ocean Counties in NJ

Rochelle Shoretz
Founder of **Sharsheret**, a national non-profit organization supporting women and families facing breast and ovarian cancer

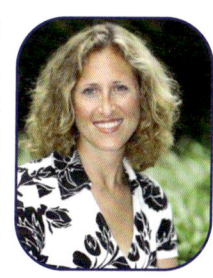

Both women had their own personal dream of creating something unique for cancer patients. Having championed their dreams to fruition, Beth and Rochelle each leave behind a legacy... caring organizations that, to this day, continue to provide care, knowledge, comfort, support, and hope to thousands of patients and their families.

Foreword

Over the years, **Sharsheret** has been proud to share **Butterfly Kisses and Wishes on Wings** with thousands of women and families across the country who come to us looking for support around talking about cancer with their children. We've heard from them how this special story has helped open the door to a tough conversation, and how it made that dialogue so much easier.

When the opportunity arose to partner with Ellen and Nanci to update and reprint their latest edition of **Butterfly Kisses and Wishes on Wings**, we jumped at the chance to help get this resource into the hands of even more children and families who need it most. Each child is different, each family is unique, and each story has its own cast of characters with their own experiences. Use this resource in the way that feels most comfortable for you. Please know that you're not alone; **Sharsheret**, and all the resources listed in the **Butterfly Kisses** resource guide and on the website, are here to help you and your children on this journey.

We hope you find this book helpful and comforting.

Elana Silber, MBA
Executive Director, Sharsheret

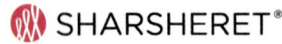

**Sharsheret would like to thank the Allergan Foundation,
for their generous support in the printing of this new edition of
Butterfly Kisses and Wishes on Wings**

Dear Readers,

The text of **Butterfly Kisses* and Wishes on Wings** was originally written as a gift for my cousin Nanci Hersh, an award-winning artist, to help her find the right words to explain her cancer diagnosis to her then 3-year-old and 5-year-old boys. Two years later, and finally in remission - along with some gentle nudging on my part, Nanci agreed to illustrate the text I had written for her boys.

Once our endeavor was completed, we realized that **Butterfly Kisses and Wishes on Wings** had become much more than a simple story. Through clear, candid text, and Nanci's exquisite illustrations, it had evolved into a resource that could be used to educate and support many other children around the world who are facing the cancer of a loved one.

We are pleased that you have chosen our book to help guide you as you teach a child about cancer. We hope our words and pictures will foster an honest and open dialogue between you and the child listening or reading along. Additionally, we hope that you will see the magic that **Butterfly Kisses and Wishes on Wings** has in bringing children to a clearer understanding of cancer, and the realization that they have great power within themselves to be an active and integral part of their loved one's cancer journey.

With butterfly wishes,
Ellen McVicker

P.S. We offer many wonderful resources for children and their families on our website.
Please visit us at **www.butterflykissesbook.com**, or contact the author directly at (303) 589-2099.
For additional support, **Sharsheret**, a national non-profit organization supporting women and families, can be reached at www.sharsheret.org or by calling toll free 866-474-2774.

* A butterfly kiss is a fluttering of one's eyelashes on someone's cheek ... which often makes them smile and giggle.

The other day my mom
went to the doctor.

She didn't even look sick,
but she said she had to go anyway.

I remember when she came home ...

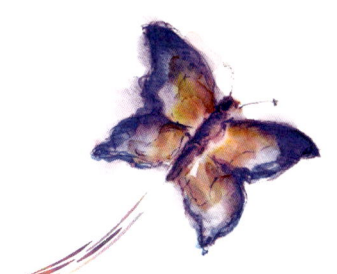

she looked worried and sad.

Later, my mom said she needed to tell me something really important.

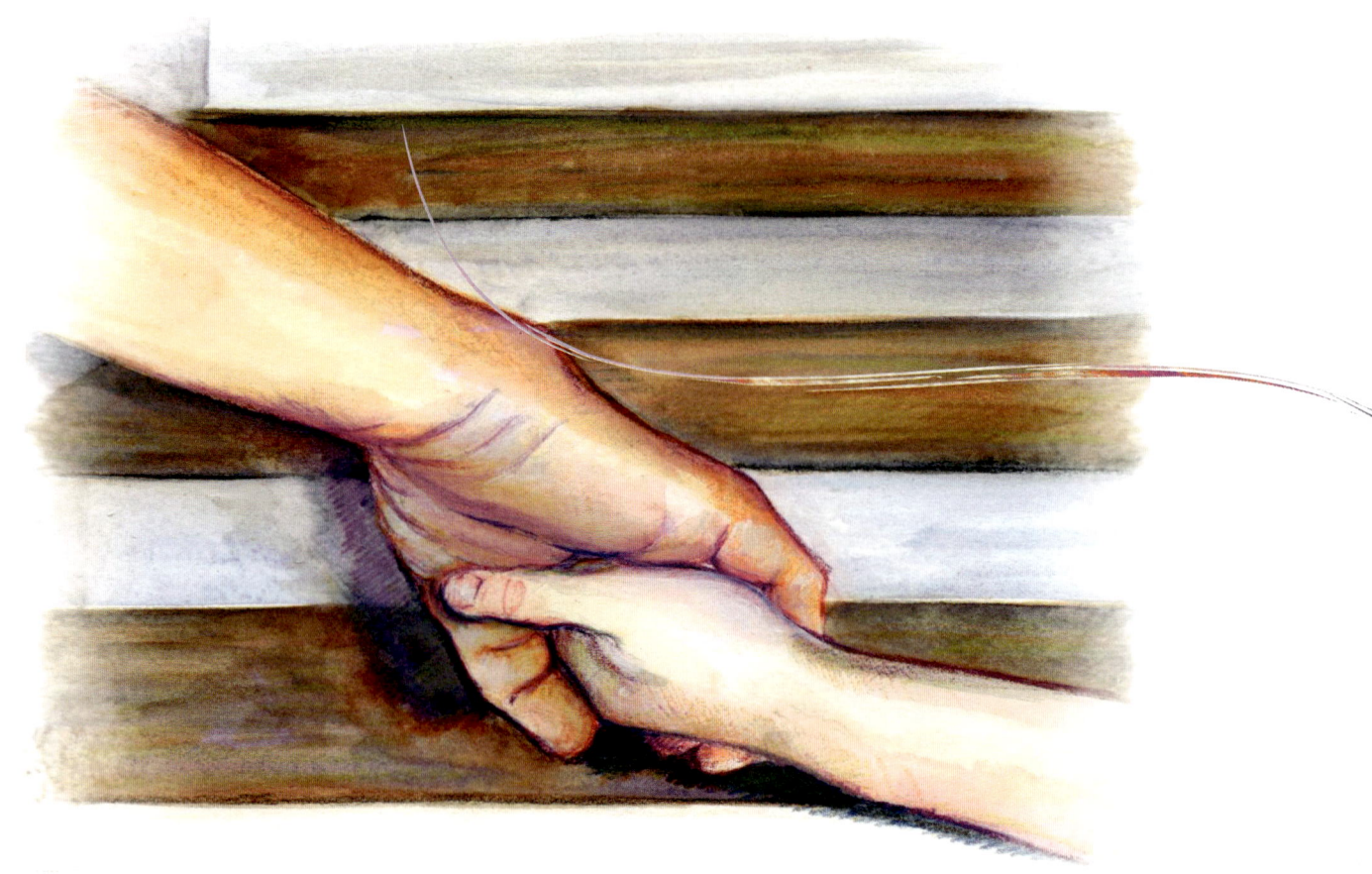

She wanted to tell me why she went to see the doctor.

But, when she started to tell me,

she looked worried and sad all over again.

Now I know why ...

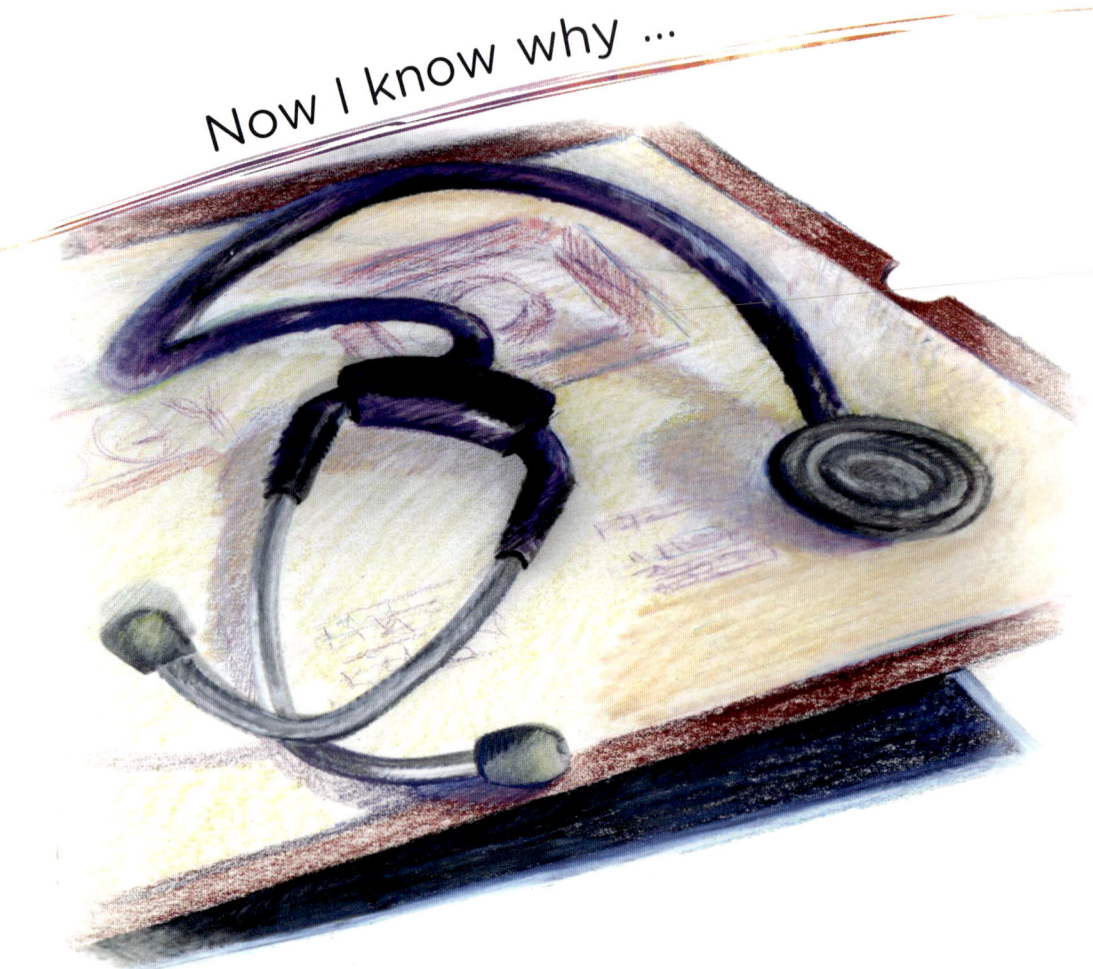

The doctor told my mom she has cancer.

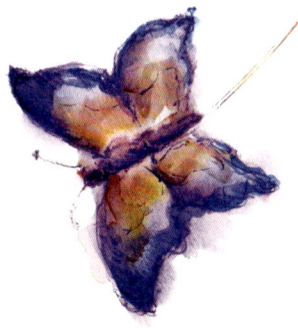

I wasn't sure what cancer was, so I asked my mom.

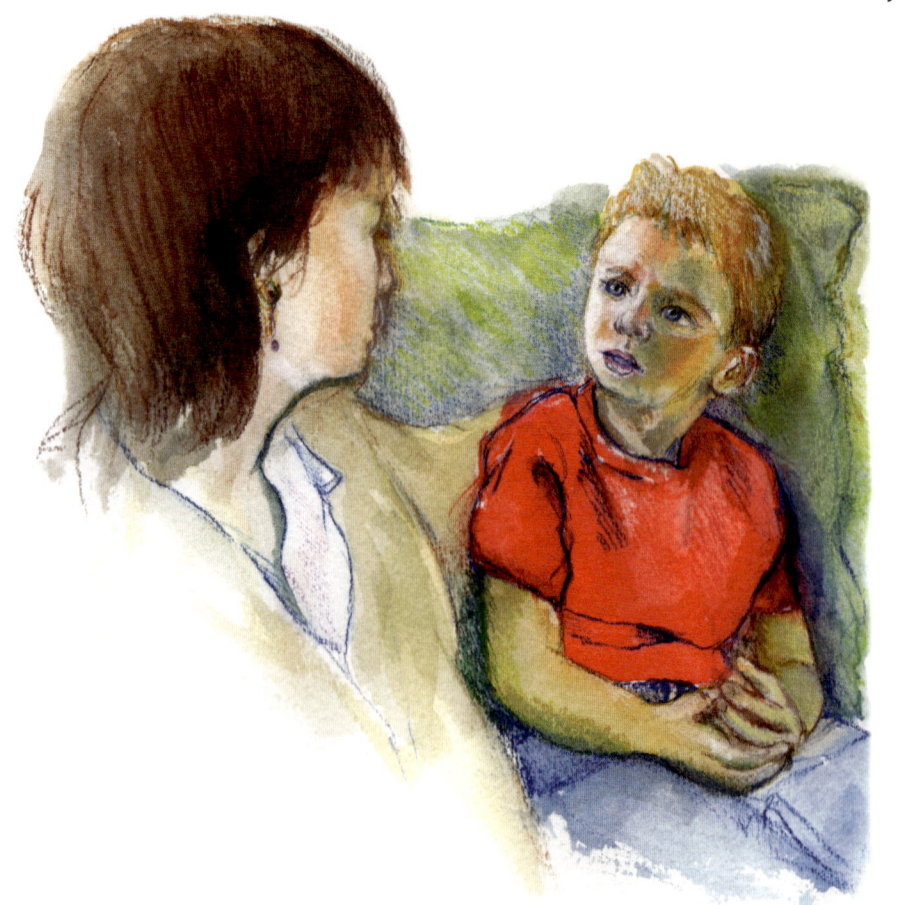

"What is cancer?"

She said it isn't like a cold or a cough or even the flu.
She said it's hard to explain.

I asked her to try anyway.

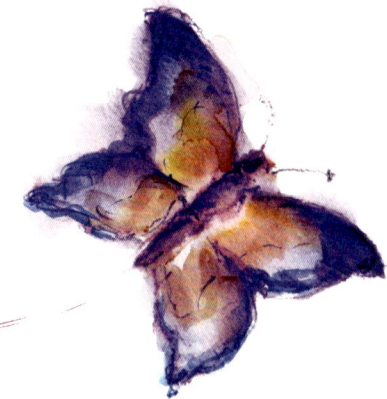

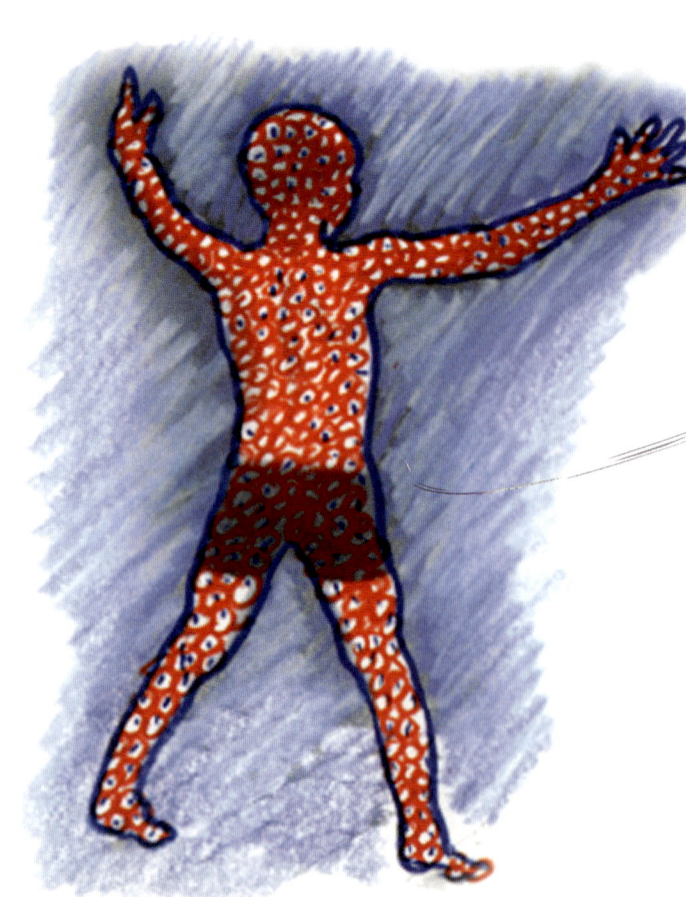

Mom said that everyone's body is made up of millions and billions of tiny cells —

so tiny, you need a microscope to see them.

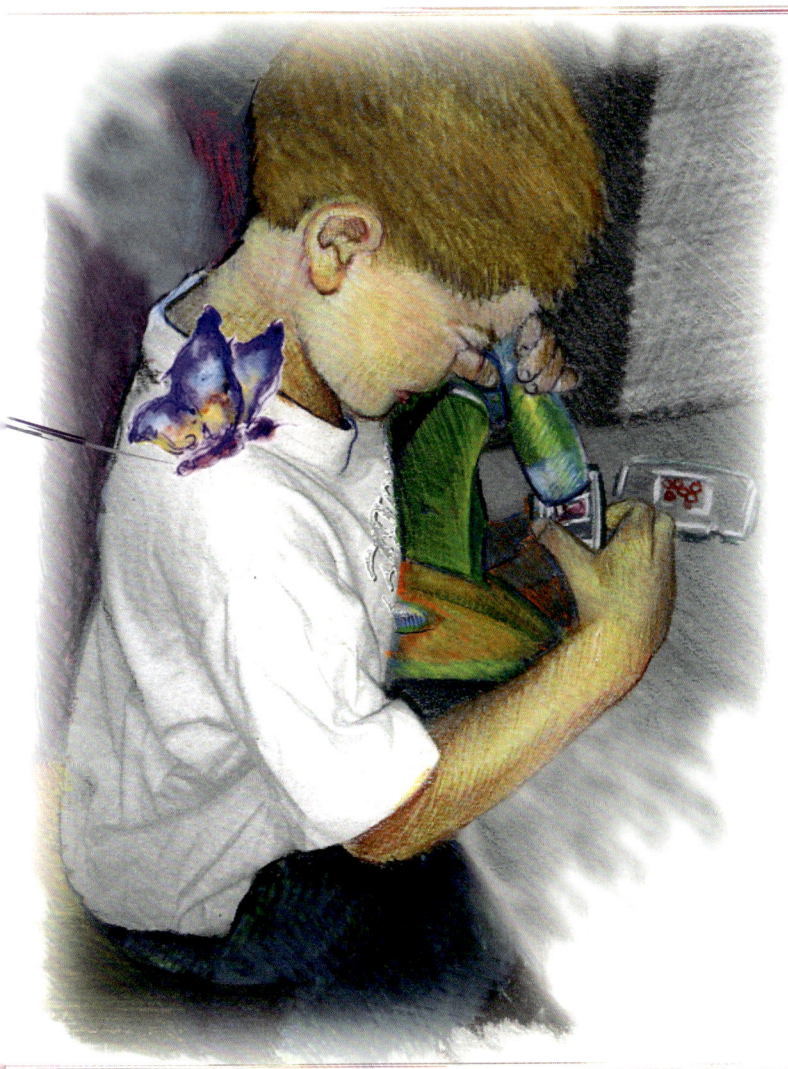

Cancer happens when some of the good cells in your body change to bad cells. No one knows why they change. They just do. It's kind of like they get sick.

Before you know it, more and more of the bad cancer cells are in your body AND they're stopping the GOOD cells from doing the job they're supposed to do.

Doctors who know all about this stuff can help people get rid of the bad cancer cells ...

and there are lots of different ways they can do it.

Some people may go to the hospital for an operation, where the doctor tries to take out all the cancer cells.

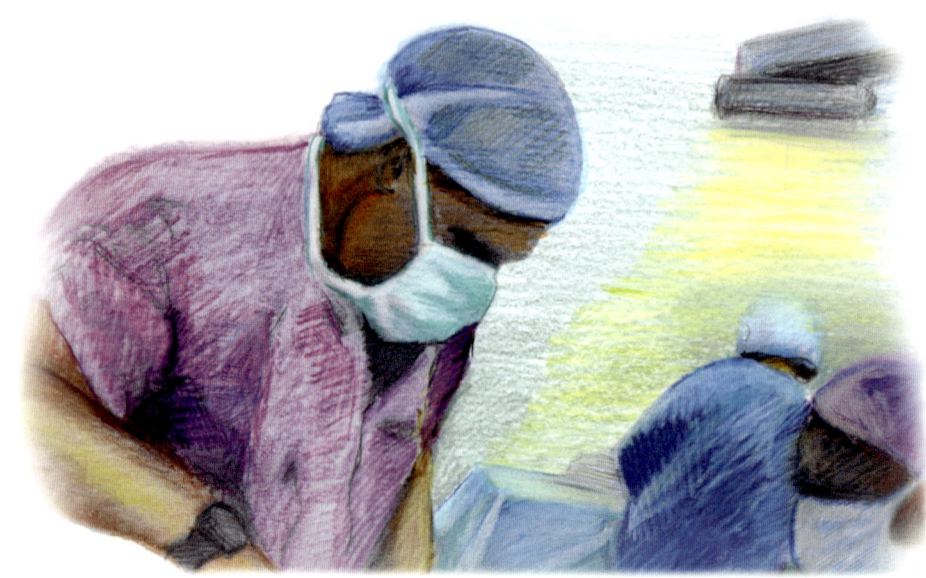

Some people may need something called radiation. Mom said that radiation is this beam of light that the doctor uses to kill the bad cancer cells.

It's kind of like my toy laser sword.

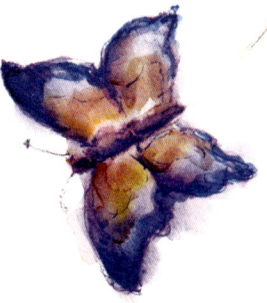

And some people may need
a special kind of medicine
called chemotherapy …
but, most people just call it "chemo."

Mom said if she has to have the chemo, it could make her tired or give her tummy aches. It may even make her hair fall out! That means she would be bald, but probably not forever. Her hair could grow back when she starts to get better.

I don't even care if
my mom does get bald.
The medicine would destroy
the cancer cells,
and that's JUST what we want!

We're not sure what
my mom needs yet.

She said the doctor will
help her decide.

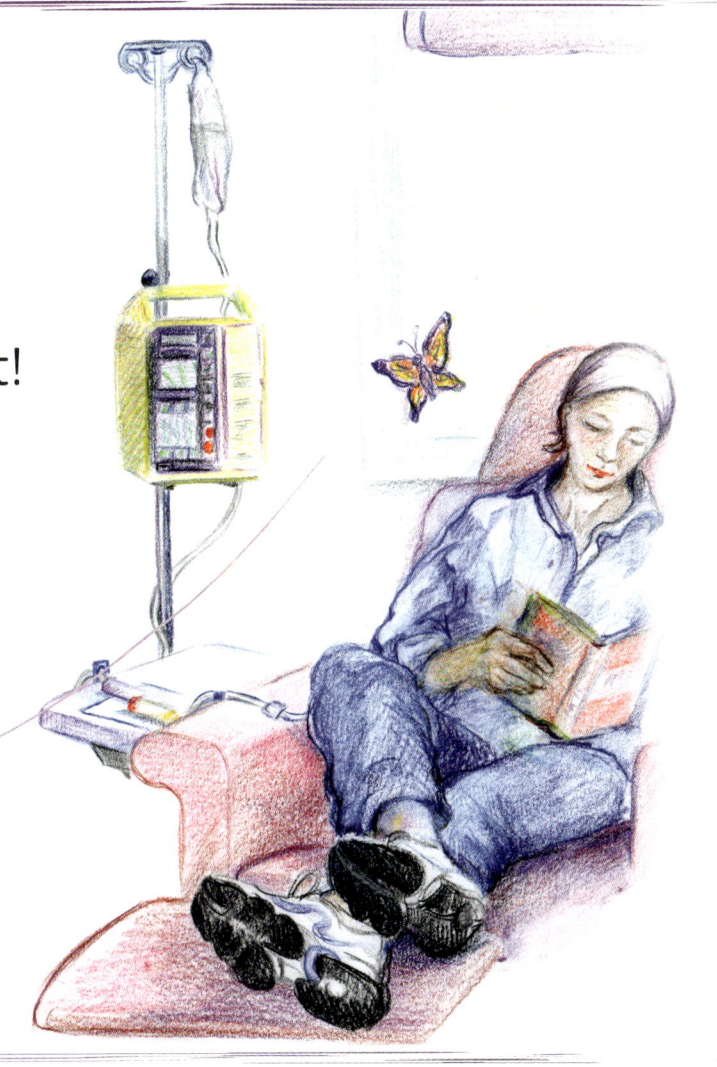

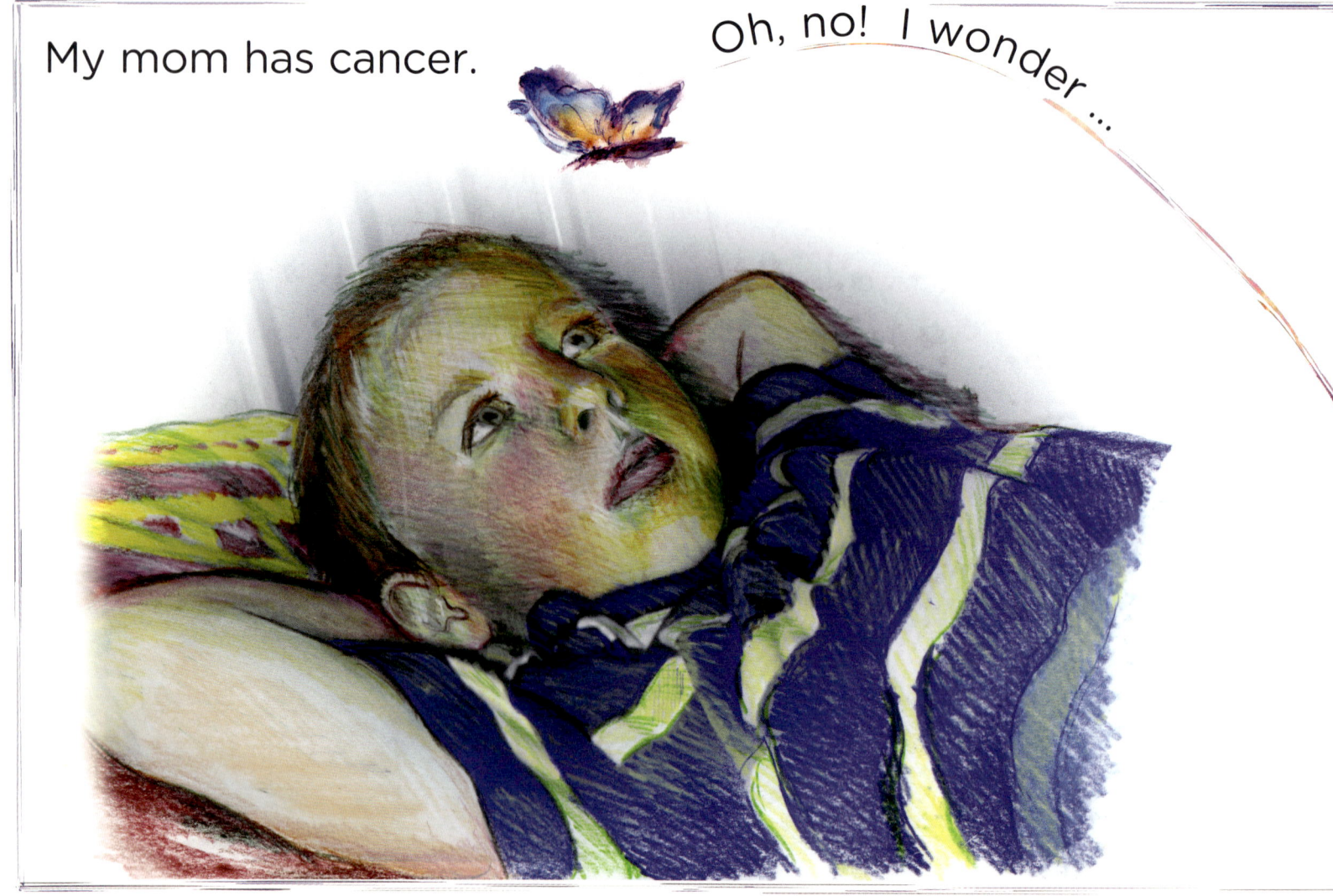

Did I do anything to make her get cancer?

If I hug and kiss my mom, will I get cancer, too?

When I asked my mom, she smiled and said I didn't do anything to make her get sick,
and that cancer is NOT contagious.

That means I can't catch cancer from her or anyone else.

She even gave me a pinkie promise.

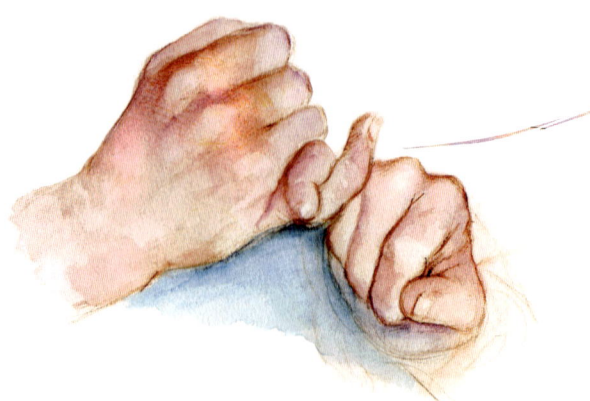

So ...

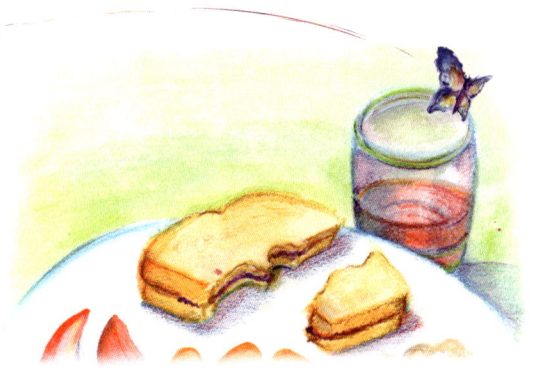

I can still take bites of her peanut butter and jelly sandwich and have a sip of her juice.

We can even share an ice cream cone. Strawberry is our favorite!

And when we cross the street, Mom can hold my hand ... just like always.

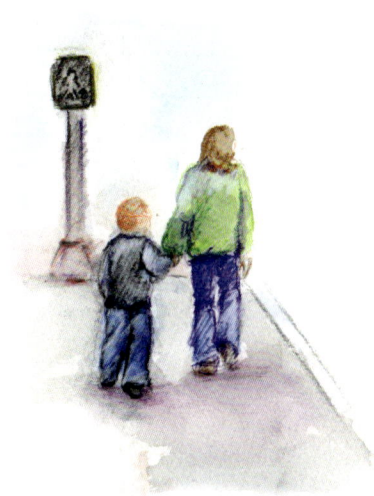

Best of all,

we can still cuddle and give lots of kisses —

butterfly kisses ... Eskimo kisses

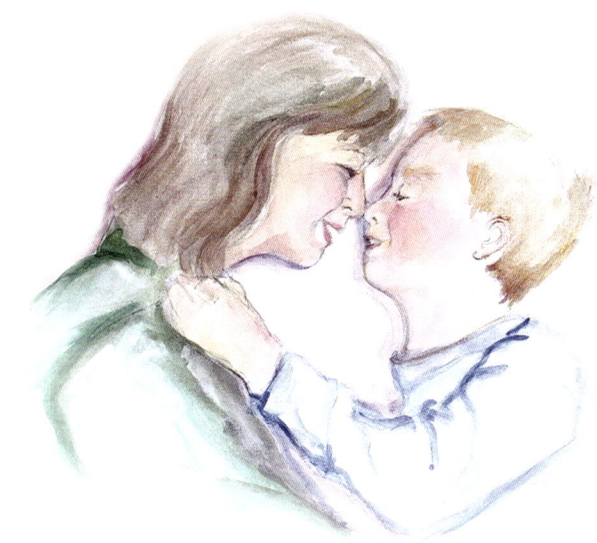

... kisses on our cheeks.

No matter what we do together, or how many kisses we give each other,
I WON'T catch her cancer.

Mom said the doctor will do everything she can to help her get better.

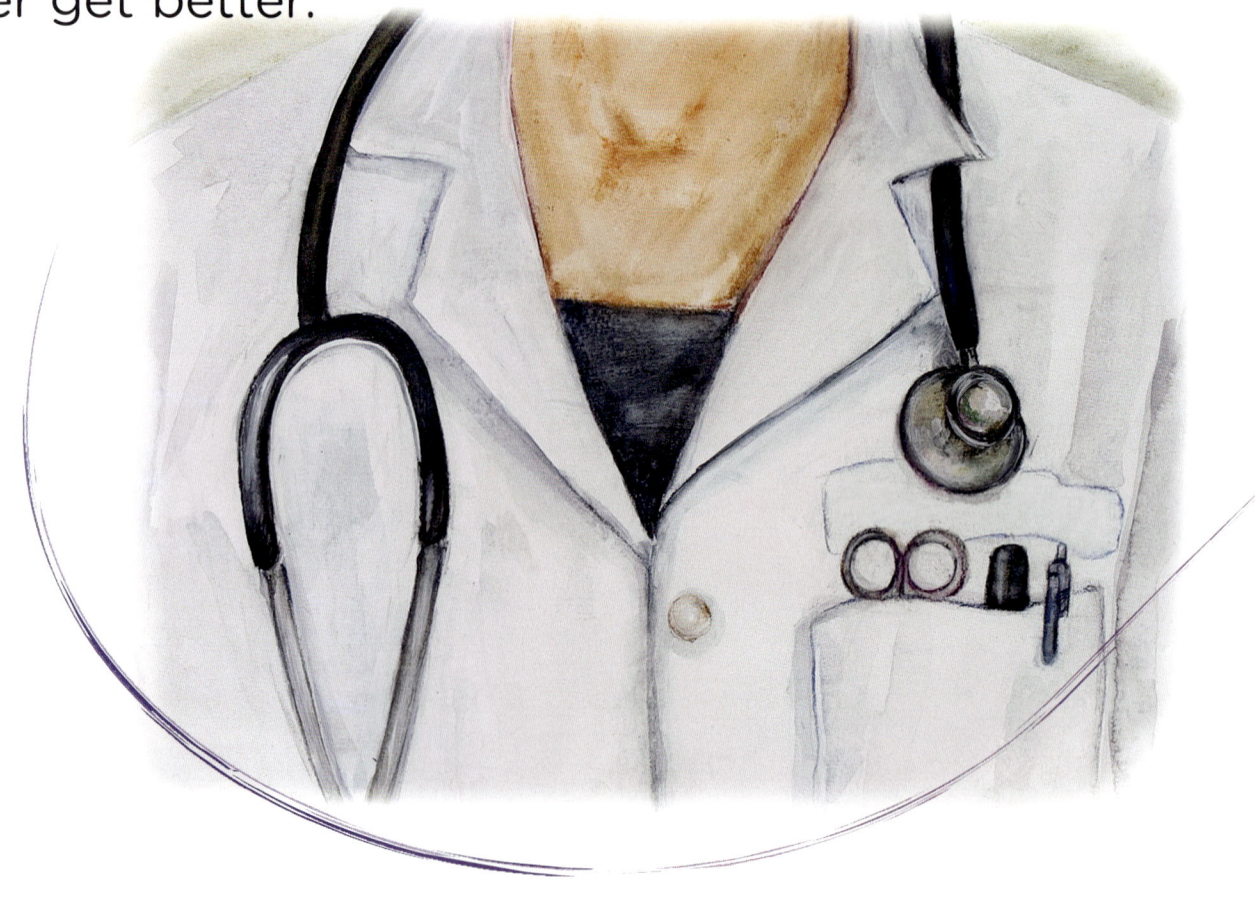

I know I can help, too!

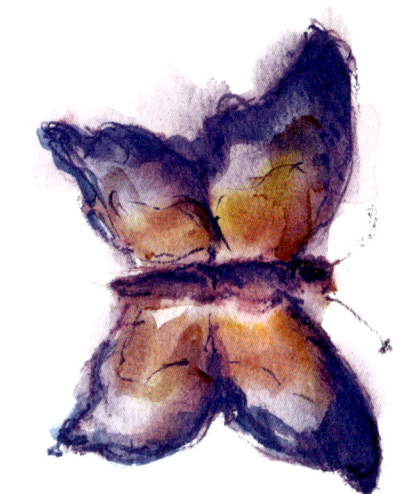

I can't make her cancer go away,
but I can do lots of other things!

I can bring her a tissue,

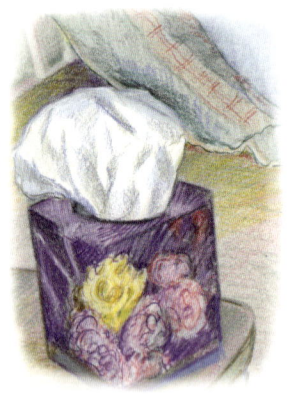

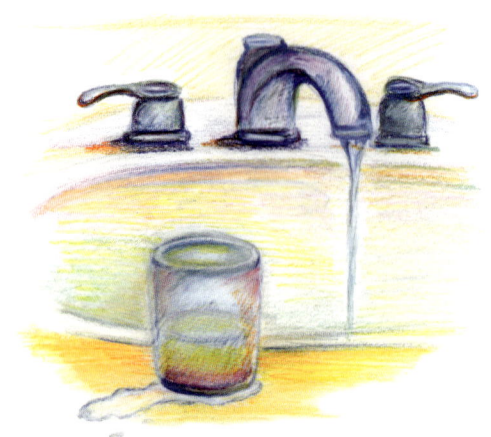

or get her a glass of water
... even if I spill a little.

When she's resting,
I can cover her toes
with a blanket
so she doesn't
get chilly.

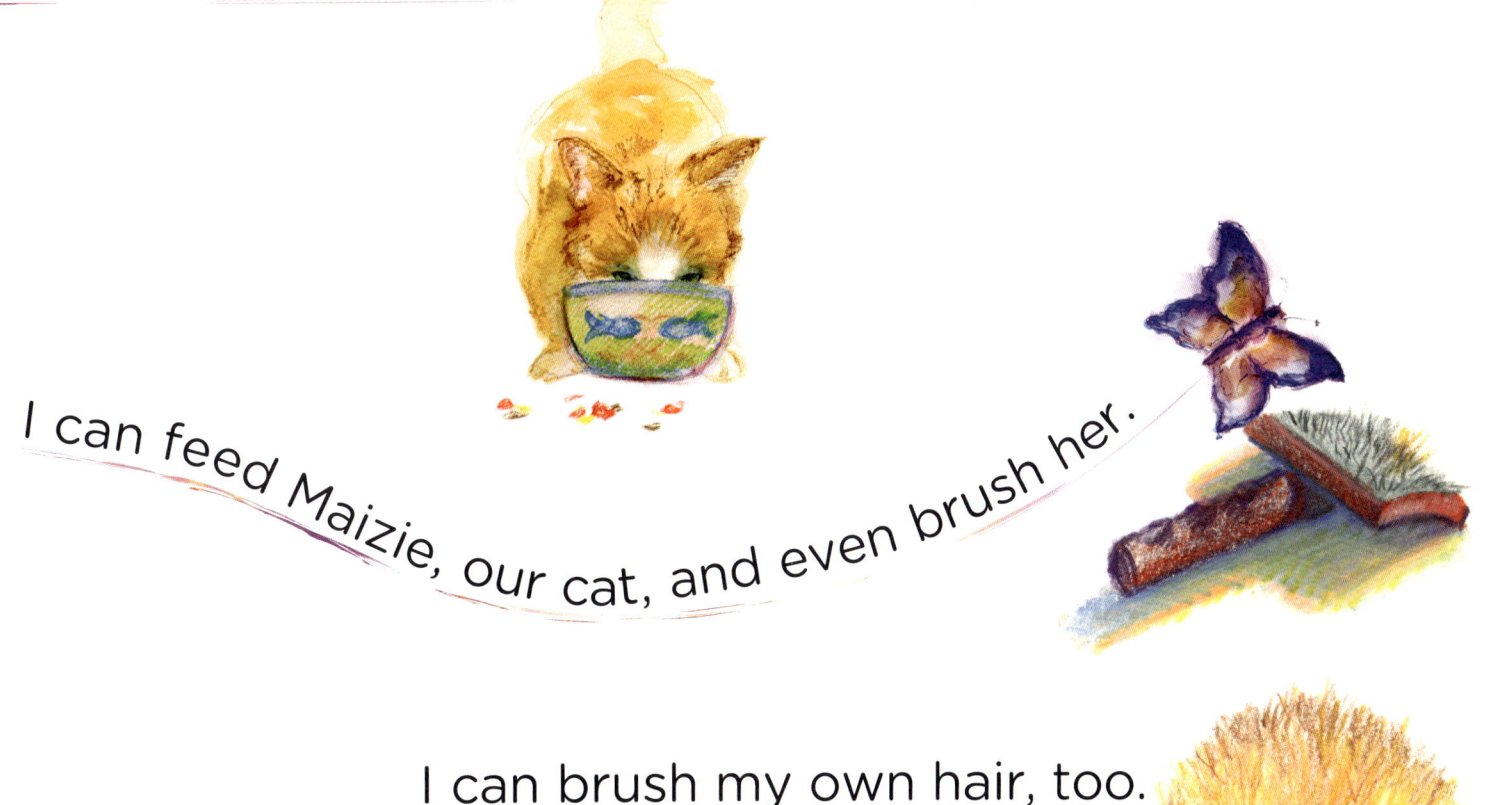

I can feed Maizie, our cat, and even brush her.

I can brush my own hair, too.
Mom laughs, because sometimes
I just use the same brush.

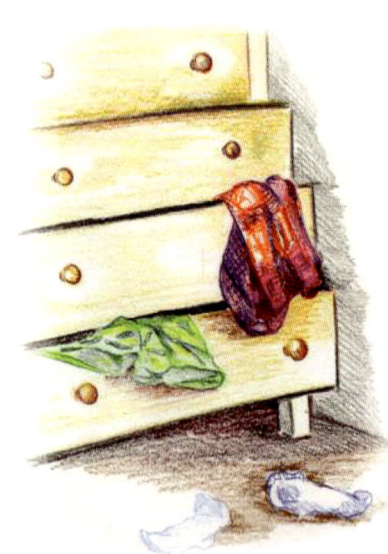

And getting dressed all by myself won't be so hard ...

So what if my clothes don't match!

If Mom needs a nap,

I'll play with my little brother so he doesn't wake her up. He can be so noisy!

But, before she takes her nap,

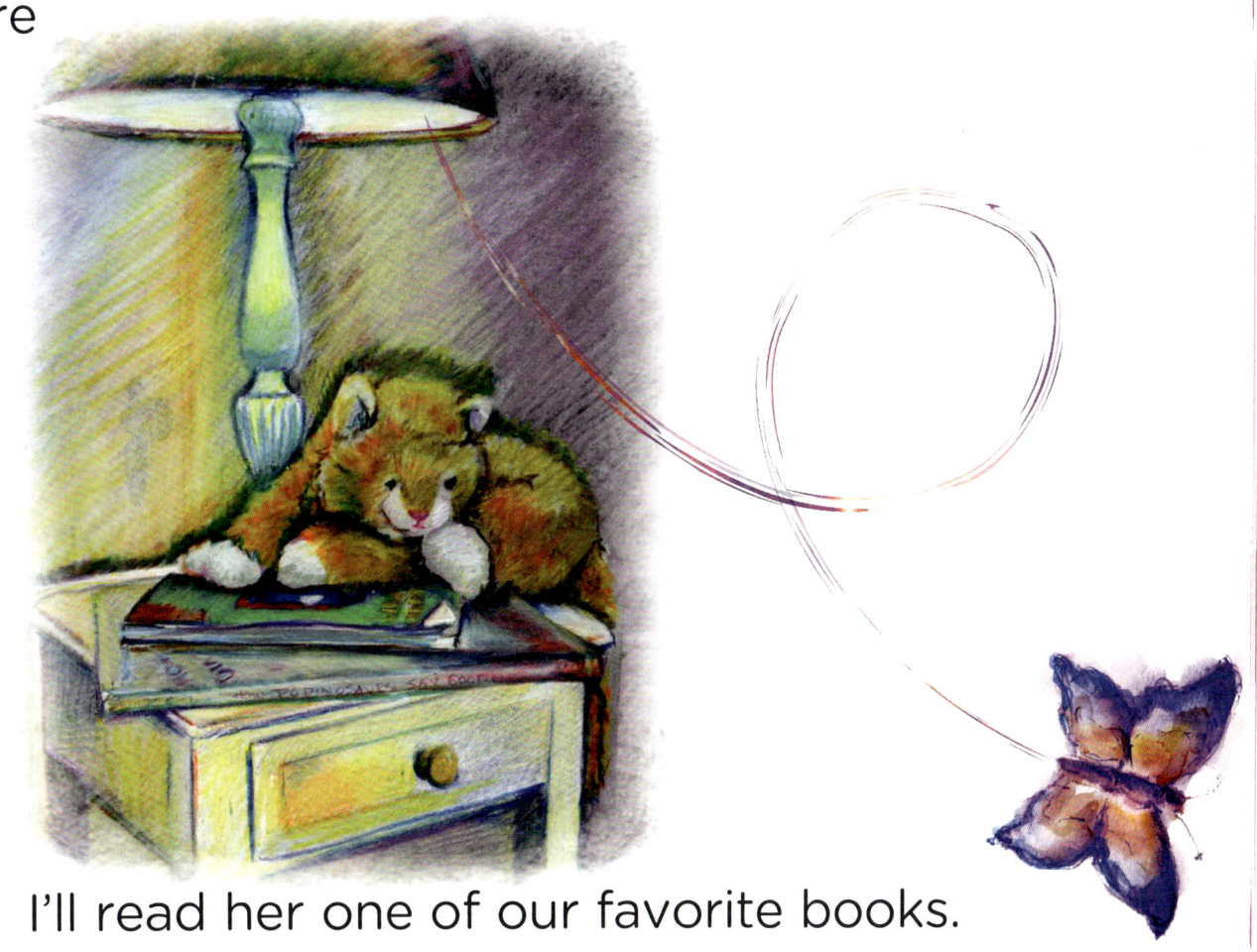

I'll read her one of our favorite books.

If Grandma or Auntie calls and asks me to spend the night,

Mom says I should go.

It would give me a break ...

and everyone needs a break now and then.

I'll even draw my mom a picture every day.

My pictures always make her smile,

and right now Mom needs a bunch of smiles!

Mom really loves it when I draw her butterflies!

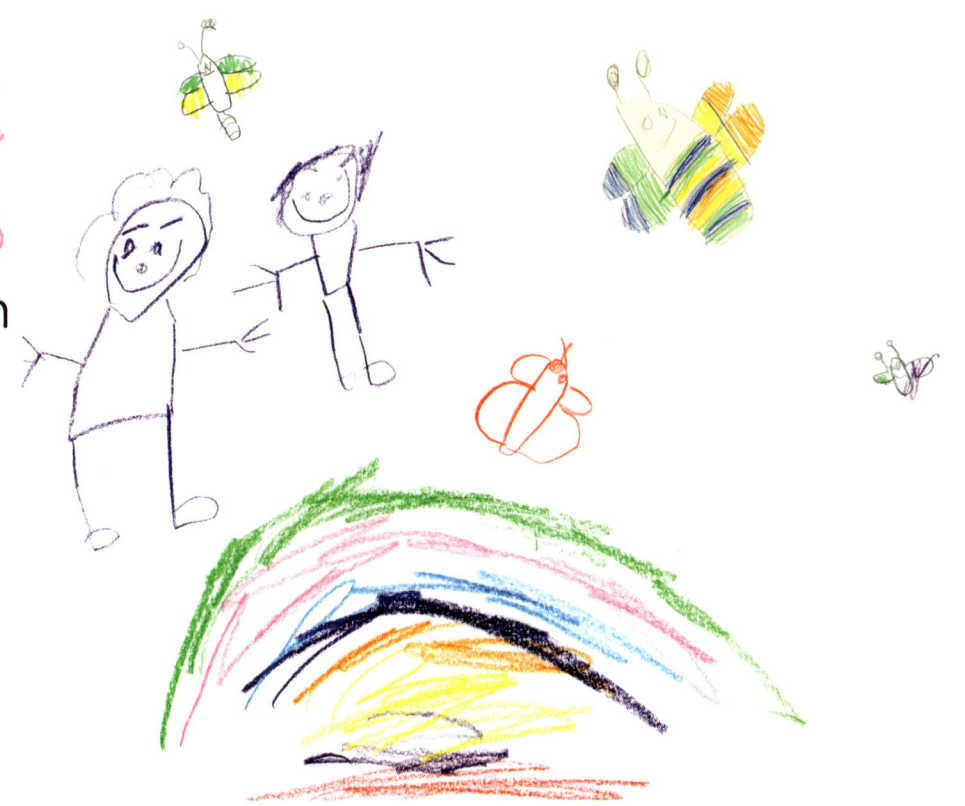

She says they remind her of our butterfly kisses,

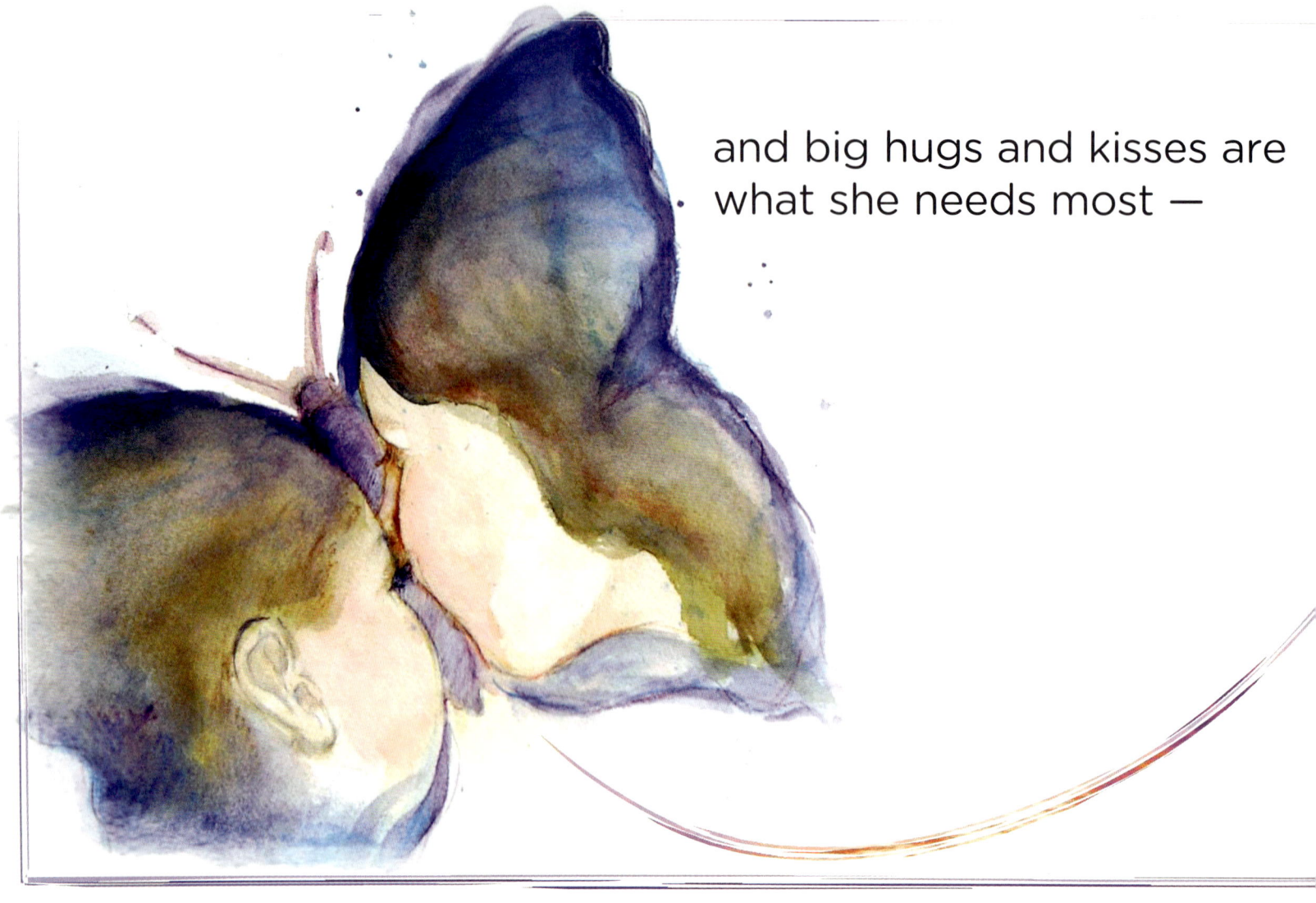

and big hugs and kisses are what she needs most —

especially my butterfly kisses!

My mom once told me that the wings of a butterfly are magical. If you watch a butterfly as it flutters its wings through the air, the butterfly will bring you good luck.

Now, more than ever, I need to be my mom's butterfly!

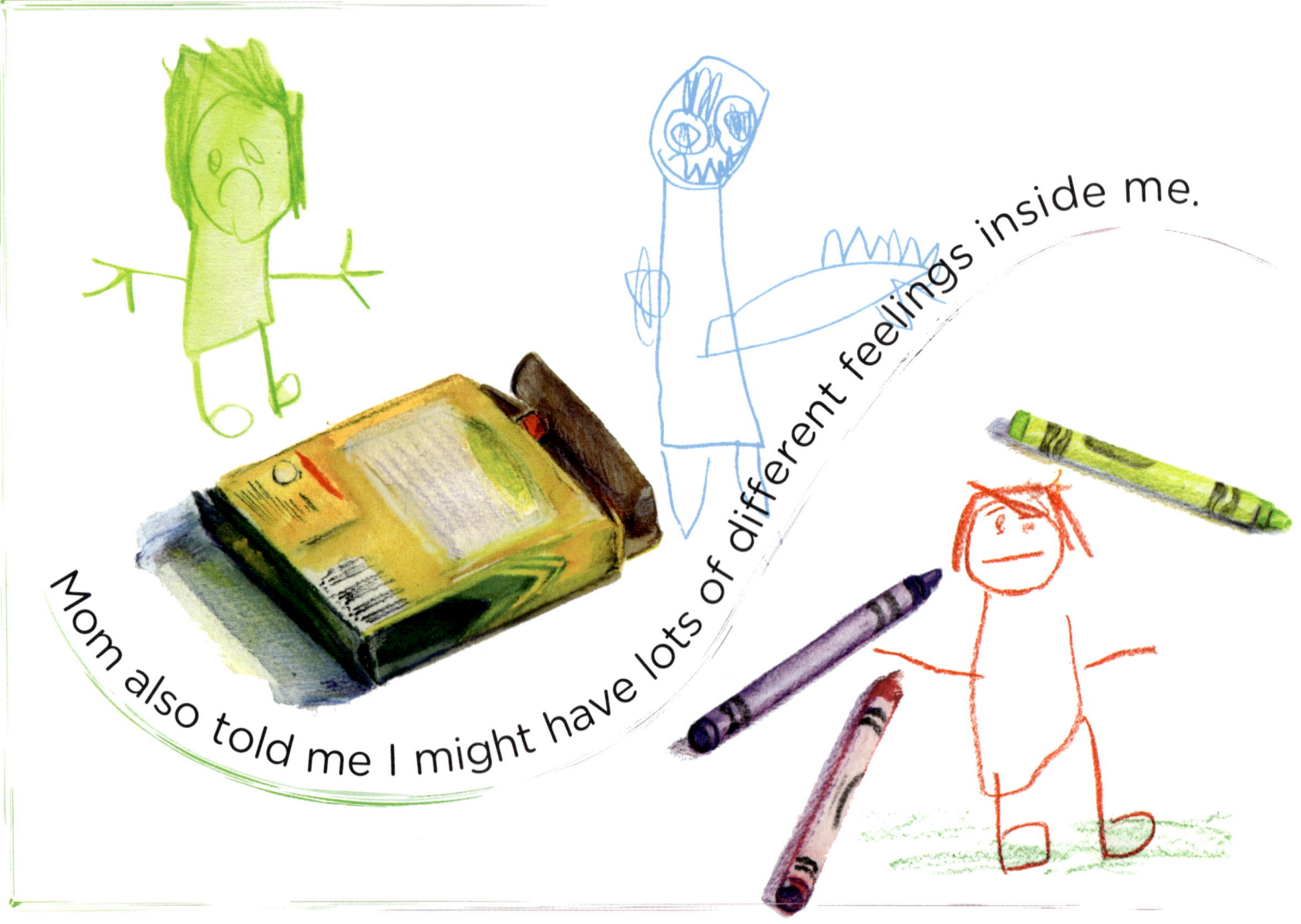

Mom also told me I might have lots of different feelings inside me.

She says some kids get SAD and feel LONELY when someone they love has cancer.

Some kids get MAD.

And then there are kids who WORRY a lot.

I'm already worried.

I worry and wonder if Mom
 will ever be okay again.

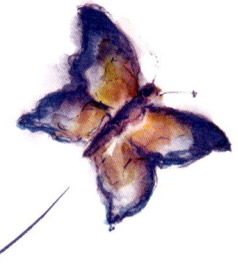

I HATE that my mom has cancer!

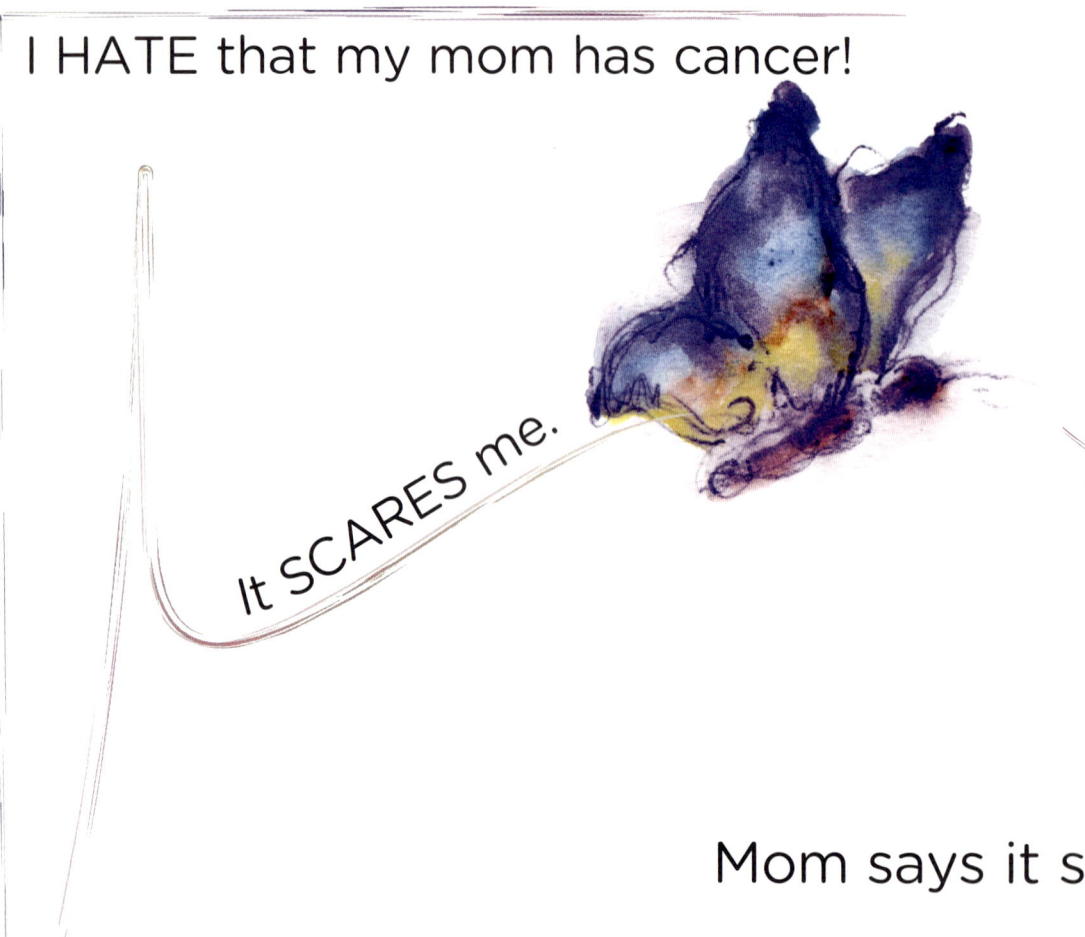

It SCARES me.

Mom says it scares her, too.

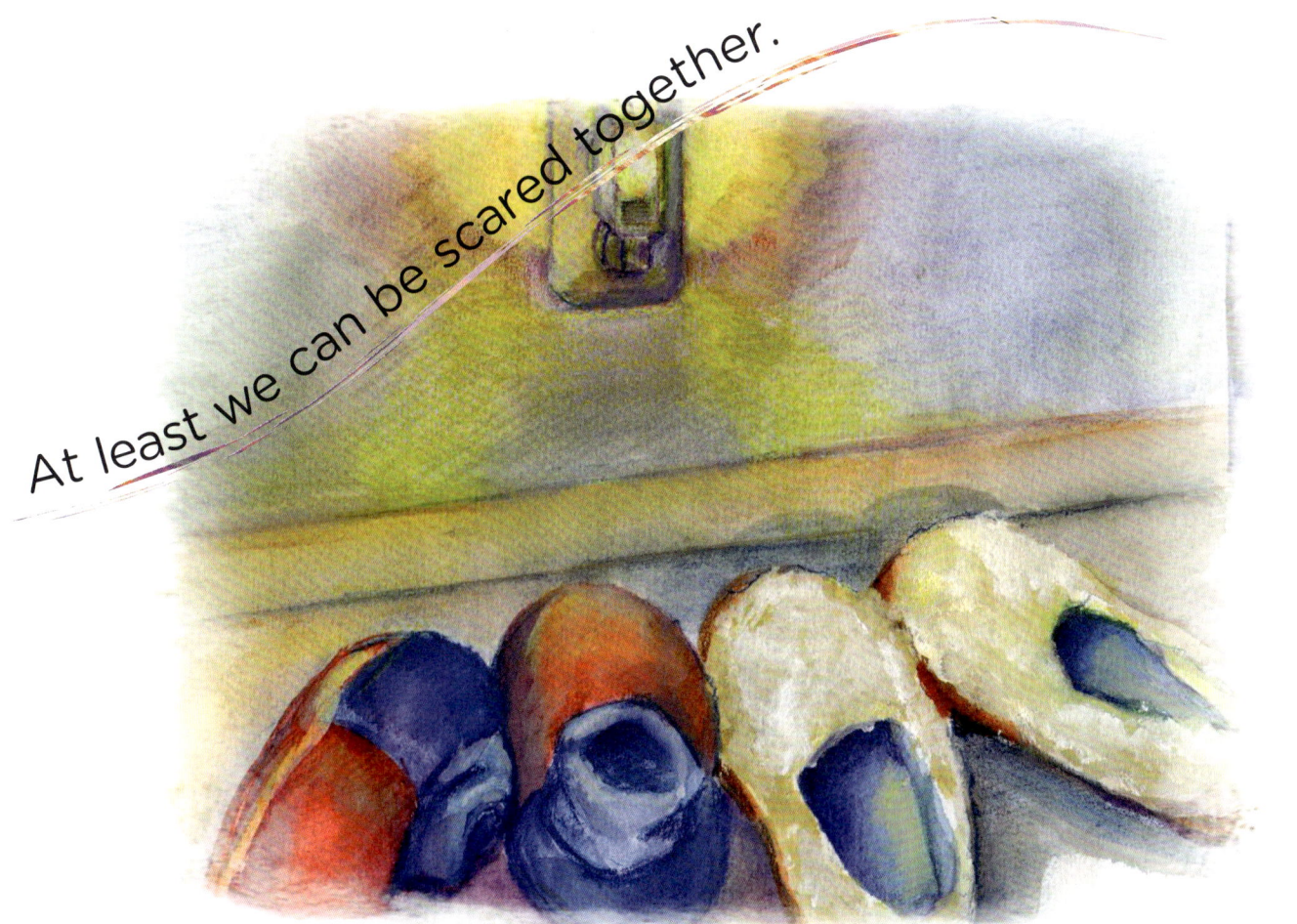

At least we can be scared together.

With all this stuff going on, Mom said it's important for me to talk about my feelings, and that it's okay to tell people that she has cancer.

That's good, because talking about things always makes me feel better inside.

I know I can talk to my dad and my best friend.

Usually I just talk to Maizie.
She's the best listener!

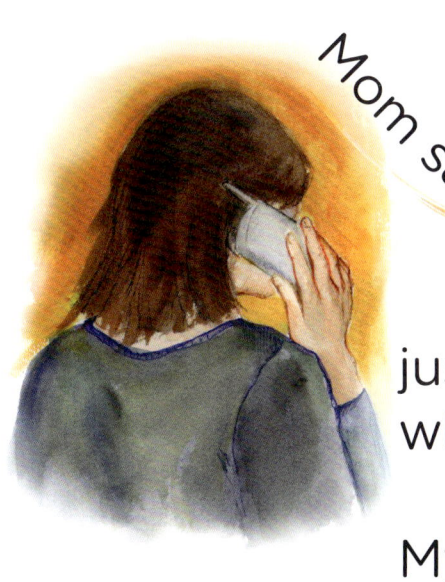

Mom said she also told my teacher all about her cancer ... just in case I start thinking about it when I'm in school.

My mom sure is smart. She's thought of everything!

But for now,

I just want to talk to my mom.

I want to give her lots of hugs and butterfly kisses, and tell her that I love her.

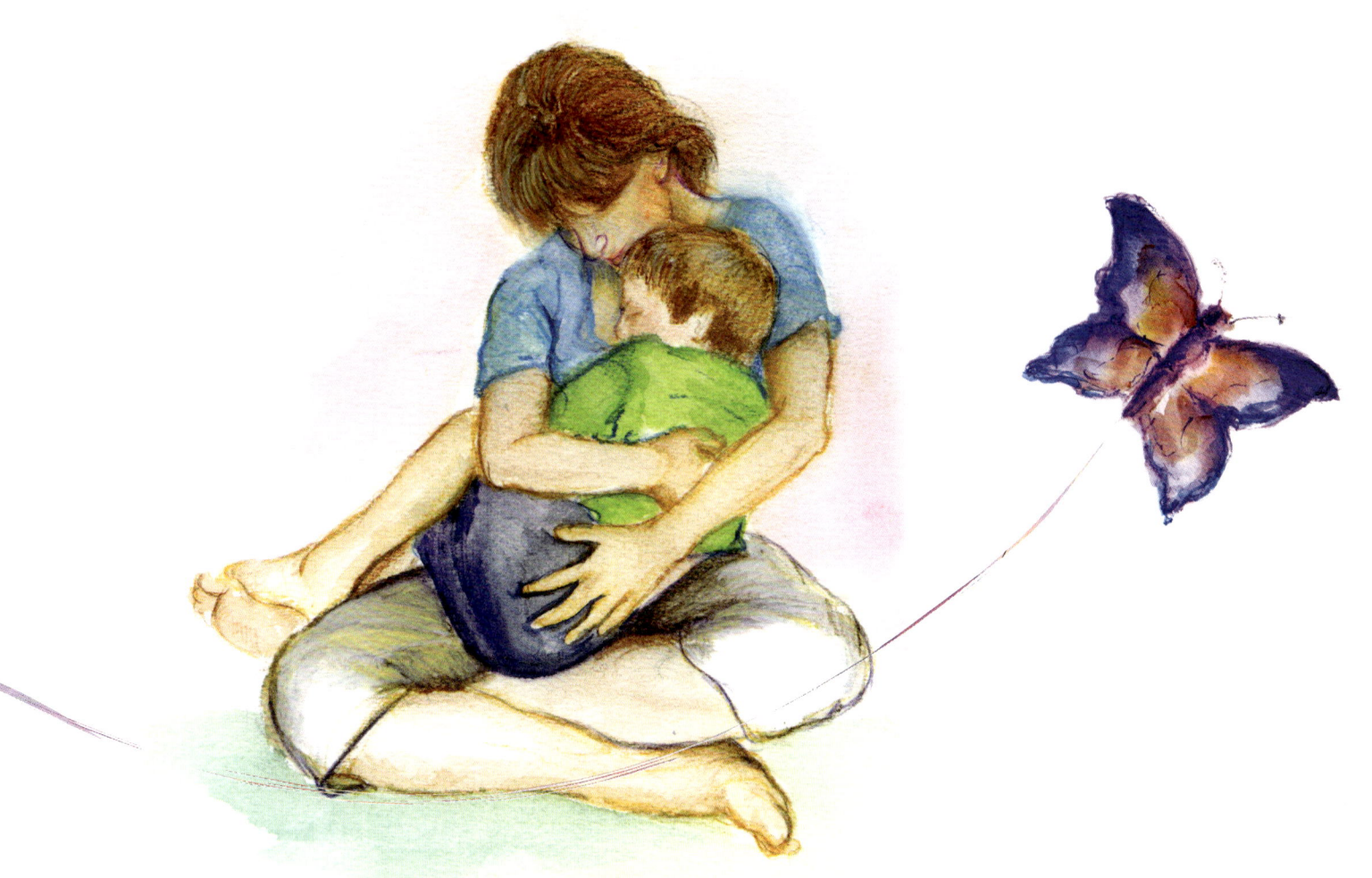

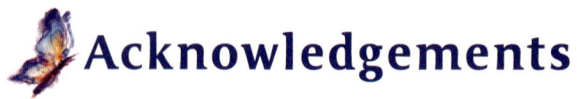 Acknowledgements

There are people who enter our lives and help us realize our potential by guiding us as we travel beyond what we sometimes believe to be our limits.
We are fortunate to have many of these people in our lives – to them we owe an abundance of thanks.

From Ellen's heart – thank you …

Nanci Hersh, my cousin, whose illustrations inspired the creation of new words and delivered the message we wanted to share
Cheryl McCallister, an angel who has guided my path professionally and spiritually
Robin Pack and **Rona Goldberg**, my sisters, my friends, and my greatest cheerleaders
Muriel Pizer, my mother, the woman who gave me my butterfly wings and taught me the importance of helping others
Tracey McVicker, my husband, and **Dustin**, **Jordan** and **Chad**, our three boys, who have been my butterflies, always traveling alongside me as I follow my dreams

From Nanci's heart – thank you …

Ellen McVicker, my cousin, whose gentle persistence in having me illustrate this story has been a source of support, healing, and love
Dr. Beth Deutch, doctor, art lover, and friend; a butterfly to so many and forever in my heart
Ellen and **Herb Hersh**, my parents whose love gave me the roots and wings to fly
Joy Dight, my mother-in-law, cheerleader and butterfly
Scott Dight, my husband, who comes from love in everything he does – and inspires me to do the same, and our children, **Griffin** and **Nate Dight**, whose love and laughter always make my heart sing

From both of us …
Fran Waldmann – a hero in our eyes for designing the book as we dreamed it should be

And in loving Memory of **Dr. Beth Deutch,** Medical Director of **HerSpace**: Breast Imaging Associates, who believed in our work from the onset, and wrote the following in our very first publication:

"How will I explain this to my children?" has impressively been the frequent first response of my young patients receiving the diagnosis of breast cancer. This speaks to how we love the children in our lives and place their well-being in front of our own. It also speaks to a need we all have in explaining cancer and illness to young children and helping them, when necessary, to be an integral part of the journey. We now recognize that to do otherwise is unhealthy. This was Nanci's concern when I delivered the news of breast cancer to her in 2002. The narrative in **Butterfly Kisses and Wishes on Wings** was her loving cousin Ellen's gift to her and her young sons. Through Nanci's beautiful and poignant illustrations, and the collaboration between cousins — the special education/kindergarten school teacher and the artist/breast cancer survivor — the gift is now for us all to cherish and use.

When Nanci first showed me this book, I cried. I cried as a mother of young children, for the clarity it brings to the young child's mind by answering the questions he may not yet be able to formulate and by calming the fears he may not yet recognize. I cried as a breast imager who daily delivers the news of breast cancer — that mothers and fathers will have one less source of anxiety with this book as a resource.

When you fly alongside the butterfly through the pages of this book, I have no doubt that you, too, will appreciate its value. It is not just for the child in the midst of a family illness. It is for all children and all parents everywhere.

And, to …
The many other wonderful, loving, and very courageous people in our lives who have dramatically been affected by cancer. Some have died; some have conquered; some have outcomes yet to be known. Each one has taught us about facing fears, taking charge, and moving on. Those who have passed away taught us about embracing life and dying with dignity.
With respect, gratitude, and our loving hearts – we thank you all.

What Our Readers Have to Say ...

"My own mother died from breast cancer when I was 8 years old. My sister, Lisa, was only five. To this day, I can so vividly remember the confusion I felt, trying to understand why our world was suddenly turned upside down and why no one wanted to talk about it. ... How I wish we had **Butterfly Kisses and Wishes on Wings** - what a gift it would have been! ... This book is precious and full of wonderful messages that are so important and will make such a difference in so many little hearts."

    Maggie O'Brien
    Middletown, New Jersey

"I believe you have captured the inner most feelings of young children. The clarity of reassurance of the child's safety and his/her remaining an integral part of the nuclear family (under the duress of illness) and being able to contribute to the parent's well being resonates in the prose. Simplicity of explanation is necessary in answering difficult questions that children pose to adults, and you have been successful in doing this with your book.

    Shirley MacPherson, Ph.D.
    Clinical Therapist/Psychologist
    Los Angeles, CA

"I read **Butterfly Kisses and Wishes on Wings** with my 6-year-old daughter. She loved the book. Her comment was 'How did the book know what I was thinking?' Your book handled the subject matter with dignity and grace."

    Dr. Sherrie Somers & daughter Chanah
    Denver, Colorado

"Your book really does address extremely well an area that many people forget about during a cancer diagnosis – the impact on the children. They are often the forgotten ones in the crisis. Making children a part of that time is so important – for everyone. I remember I used to use what I called "love therapy." I would hug my boys so tightly that I was convinced it was making me better, because I couldn't possibly imagine not being there for them. Well, it worked."

    Lorry Gaidus, Breast Cancer Survivor (12 years!)
    Upper Saddle River, N.J.

"Did you know that some of the best medicine for some diseases is love and lots of help? I learned that and other things from Mrs. McVicker's book, **Butterfly Kisses and Wishes on Wings**. If anyone wants to read something about cancer, Mrs. McVicker's book is the right way to go."

    Virginia Nystrom
    3rd grader
    Aurora, CO.

Throughout her professional life, **Ellen McVicker** has always worked in some capacity with children, parents, educators, and people who were dedicated to the mental health profession. As a master teacher in the field of special and regular education, the Director of Education for both Charter Hospital of Denver and the Colorado Children's Museum, and as Marketing Director for the Centre for Behavioral Health at Denver's Porter Memorial Hospital, Ellen would always find ways to fulfill her true life's passion ... **empowering children and their families in challenging situations.**
Today, Ellen McVicker lives in Aurora, Colorado with her husband, Tracey. Semi-retired, she continues to teach in the public schools while remaining committed to sharing the many messages from their book with children and their families.

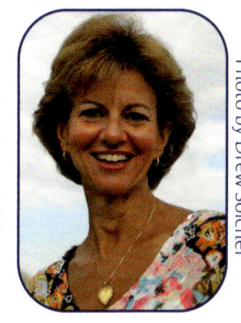
Photo by Drew Soicher

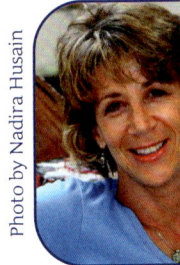
Photo by Nadira Husain

Nanci Hersh's art has always been about people and situations that are close to her heart. Following her diagnosis of breast cancer in 2002 many gifts came Nanci's way. Among these gifts were a blank sketchbook from friends and this story from her cousin. These two gifts began a journey of healing and gratitude which led Nanci to create the illustrations that have become **Butterfly Kisses and Wishes on Wings**.

Nanci is an award-winning artist, educator, and advocate for the arts. She has exhibited her work in Japan, Australia, and throughout the United States. Her work is in numerous public and private collections. Nanci Hersh lives in beautiful Chester County, Pennsylvania, with her husband Scott Dight and their two sons, Griffin and Nate. You can reach Nanci and see more of her art at **www.nancihersh.com**.

Proudly, **Butterfly Kisses and Wishes on Wings** has traveled to many parts of the world, and can be found in libraries, cancer centers, hospitals, and in the homes of many children and their families. For more information about our book, and additional resources on talking to kids about cancer, please log on to, **www.butterflykissesbook.com**. You can also reach the author at **ellenmcvicker@butterflykissesbook.com**, or by phone at 303-589-2099.

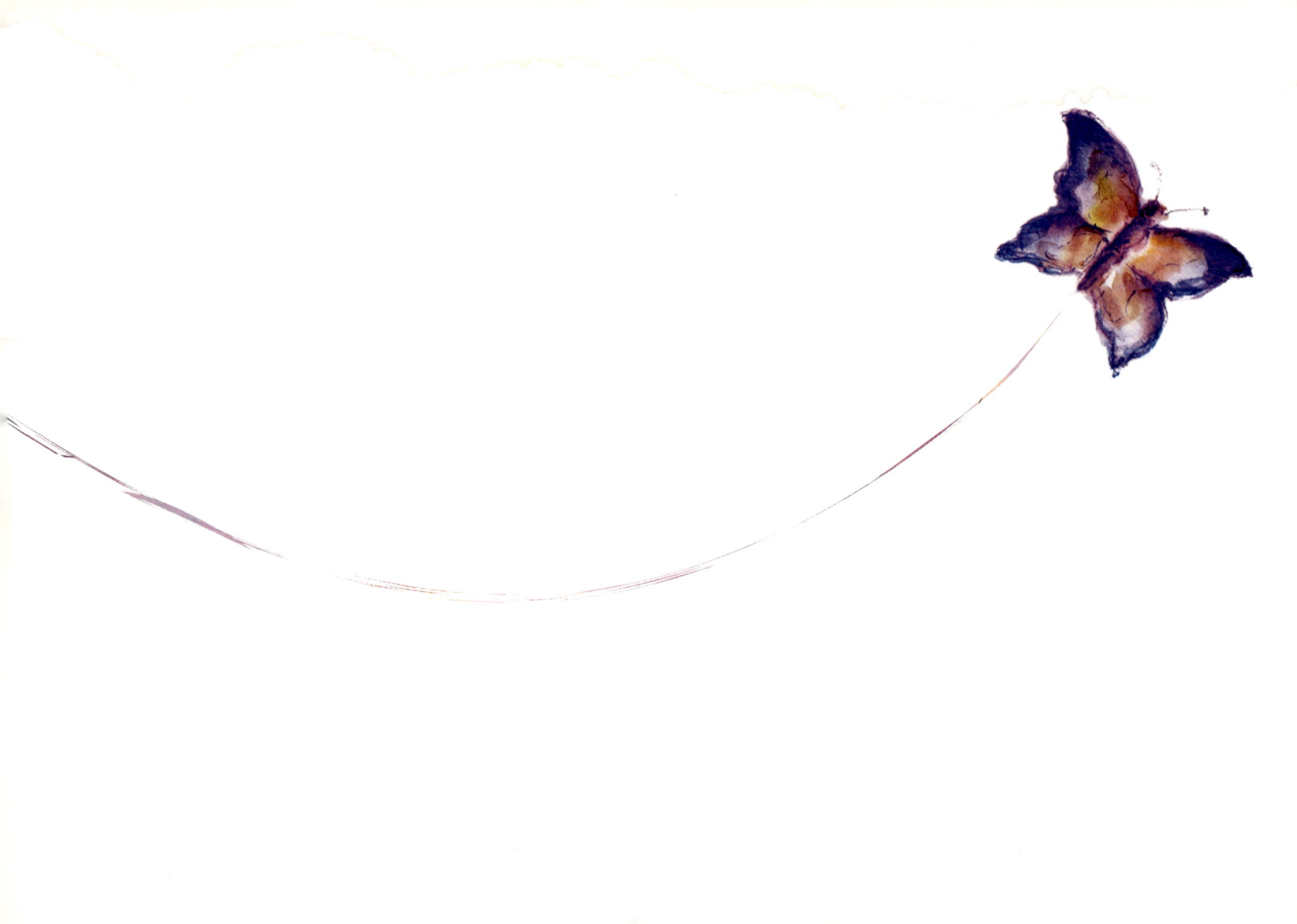